Essential Oils for Diffuser

40 Perfect Recipes for Every Day

Table of Contents

Introduction

I would like to first thank and congratulate you for downloading **"Essential Oils: Try Out 40 Perfect Diffuser Recipes for Every Day!"** You may be surprised to learn that at least 47% of the adult population will have to deal with a headache at least once a year. One of the most common disorders of the nervous system is the headache, that for many can be very painful and disrupt their way of lives. Often people suffer the discomfort of headaches without finding any true relief, that is until they discovered using a diffuser and essential oils.

Many people have tried other means in trying to get rid of headaches, more people are looking for more natural solutions rather than depending on synthetic drugs that have many bad side effects with them. So now you can go through this guide and hopefully find solutions that are going to work for you and your loved ones.

Essential oils are not something that have been discovered recently, in fact they have been around for many decades. They have been traced back to 18,000 B.C.E. There was a few cave paintings in the area of Dordogne, France these suggest the use of medicinal and herbal plants. Depending on the people's religious, or cultural beliefs the consumption of oils varied, also the beliefs and health purposes for them varied also.

History shows that the Egyptians were one of the first people to use essential oils for beauty treatments, health purposes, along with the preparation of foods, and religious and cultural activities. Often exchanged for gold was cinnamon, myrrh, sandalwood, and Frankincense as they were much sought after during this era.

Many countries such as Greece, India and China used essential oils as part of therapeutic massage, aromatherapy, and Ayurvedic purposes as well. During the dark ages oils were mainly used for their anti-bacterial and fragrant properties.

During modern times the wonderful healing powers of essential oils were actually discovered by a French Chemist, Rene-Maurice Gattefosse in 1937. He was tending to a person with a badly burnt hand and he used lavender oil to heal the hand. This was only the beginning and later on Dr Jean Valnet, a French contemporary, became famous due to his develops that he made in the use of aromatherapy practices where he introduced essential oils to injured soldiers during World War II. The growing industry surrounding essential oils is due to researchers and medical practitioners studying them and experimenting with the benefits of essential oils in regards to health and wellness benefits.

World wide essential oils are sought by many for their widely believed healing agents in many remedies that treat ailments from skin conditions to cancer. Amongst the masses aromatherapy, a branch of alternative medicine has gained much popularity with essential oils playing a major part in this treatment as aromatic plant extracts and essential oils are used for cosmetic and healing purposes. The essential oils are volatilized in a carrier oil and used for massages, and added to nebulizer to be diffused into the air or heated with a candle flame or used in burning incense.

Basic Facts About Essential Oils

There are some countries that have imposed regulations for the use of essential oils it is still popularly used for fringe medicine and popular natural remedies. Many researchers have claimed that some essential oils may have the ability to prevent the transmission of certain drug resistant strains of pathogen, specifically Candida, Staphylococcus, and Streptoco.

Essential oils can be used for numerous purposes and they may be applied as a single oil or as a complex blend. When it comes to the administration of essential oils this can be done by three different methods: diffused aromatically, applied topically or taken internally as dietary supplements which should be recommended by a physician.

Caution!

There are many essential oils that can be hazardous if they are taken by mouth due to their high concentration which might give a person the feeling of burning that is then followed with salivation.

You should never apply undiluted essential oils to your skin as this could create sensitization. It could end up resulting in a bad rash, itchy skin or in extreme cases it could lead to respiratory issues or anaphylactic shock. If you are allergic to an essential oil you are most likely going to remain permanently sensitized to the oil, even if it is diluted. You could also develop similar conditions using other essential oils.

If you are uncertain about the dosage for an essential oil it is best to speak with someone that is well-experienced in dealing with essential oils.

Keep These Facts in Mind

- You should never apply essential oils directly to your skin until they have been diluted first. Aromatherapy practitioners may make some exceptions, but these decisions need to be made by someone that is not a novice. Someone that when it comes to applying and using essential oils performs this in a safe and responsible manner.

- When it comes to you purchasing your essential oils make sure you are getting pure and recommended oils, and follow the label instructions on how to store it properly.

- You may have an allergic condition when using some essential oils for the first time. You can prevent this from being wide spread over your body by first doing a skin patch test to see how your skin reacts to the particular essential oil that you are using.

- You should never apply essential oils in or around your eye area or on open and sore wounds. These oils should not be used during pregnancy and should be avoided if you suffer from certain conditions such as epilepsy and asthma.

- You should never take essential oils internally unless you are prescribed to do so by a consultant.

- Do not allow your children to touch or play around with essential oils. Because some essential oils smell good a small child may attempt to drink them.

- Keep in mind that essential oils are flammable and must be stored out of reach of children.

- Try to handle essential oils like you would any other medicine, make sure that it is kept in an appropriate and safe place.

Do Not Use on Your Pets

You may have read in publications that using essential oils on your pets is okay, well they are not, your pets cannot handle the potency of the oils. Oils that are highly safe for us humans can end up being highly toxic for our pets. Oils such as Lavender, Terpenes, and Thyme can cause liver and or kidney failure in cats.

Some articles have even mentioned that Lavender and Thyme are wonderful to help get rid of fleas and ticks. Do not use essential oils on your pets, Tansy has been poisonous to both horses and cattle. If they have accidental exposure look for signs that your pet is in distress. My dog has licked my arm where I had essential oil blend and she was fine, but let us not take unnecessary risks with our pets health.

Many controversial disagreements over the use of aromatherapy internally is still up for debate. The National Association of Holistic Aromatherapy discourages Aromatherapists from using essential oils internally unless they have special training in which to do that. The security of the internal issue is currently being explored.

Essential oils are becoming more and more relevant in Traditional Medicine as scientists are beginning to agree that the fundamental materials have value because of their wide assortment of components. Modern medicine is leaning more towards holistic approaches to wellness they are driving a new discovery of essential oil wellbeing applications.

You can help yourself from developing ailments like colds by taking different Eucalyptus essential oils to help protect you against catching a cold by building up a protection barrier for you. You can change your mood through a Fragrance, the summer time is alive with life and the lovely fragrant smells of flowers and herbs floating through the air.

To keep the air fresh in your home try to stay away from using Plugin air fresheners. These contain harmful chemicals, which can cause damage when they are inhaled. Instead invest in an essential oil diffuser this will prove to be a much healthier choice.

Why not add some dried lavender to a vase and place it beside your headboard, this will help relax you so that you may fall asleep with ease.

What Are You Going to Use Essential Oils For?

If you are looking for essential oils just to use as a form of aromatherapy or to add a nice fragrance to your home then you can choose a fragrance or food grade type which is not very expensive. These are often distilled using synthetic solvents and do not contain pure essential oils. Whether they are 100% pure is highly unlikely for this type or grade of essential oils.

You need to understand that this grade of essential oils to not carry any kind of therapeutic value. These you can purchase just about anywhere. If on the other hand you are looking to use the essential oils as some type of remedy then you need to go for a 100% pure therapeutic grade of oils.

This grade of oils carry solvents and come tested meeting the required standards. These grade of oils are very expensive and are only supplied by a few quality suppliers.

Make sure to go to the best quality supplier that has created a good name for themselves on the good quality of therapeutic essential oils that they offer. Do some research to identify the best supplier of therapeutic essential oils. It is best to play it safe before you hand over the money for your essential oils.

How Long Does Essential Oils Last?

The shelf life of essential oils will depend on multiple factors. For example any aspect that will cause the oils to become destabilized will result in deterioration of the duration.

The atmosphere around the essential oils such as temperature, sunlight exposure, and air-conditions will have an effect on essential oils even when they are kept in the best conditions. Some oils can deteriorate quickly while others may last you a lifetime.

Check out the storage conditions when you are investing quite a bit of money when buying therapeutic grade oils. When the oils are in proper storage containers this will help keep the oils preserved and keep them so that they will give a good impact. You should always store your oils in a cool dark place where there is no sunlight and no influence of weather and temperature affecting the oils.

Many people are curious about essential oils but they are not sure how they can use or apply them. The best way that you can start to benefit immediately from essential oils is to disperse them into the air of your home using a diffuser.

Diffusing essential oils into your home air will only benefit you and your loved ones due to the fact that they have proven antibacterial and antiviral actions; they can destroy and ruin microbes in the air.

You can disinfect the air supply of your home using a diffuser for antiviral/antimicrobial activity and immune support. Using a nebulizing diffuser can help cut down on costs so that you can evaporate therapeutic doses of essential oils in your home environment.

Storing Essential Oils

The best place to store essential oils is in dark colored glass bottles as they will offer protection to the oils. You do not want to leave the bottles out in the sunlight as they will heat up and this will increase the process of deterioration of your essential oils.

Do not store your essential oils in a plastic bottle, as this highly concentrated oil will eat into the plastic and decay in no time at all. Make sure to always tighten the cap securely after using the oils or they will evaporate in seconds.

What a Diffuser Does

What a diffuser does is to break the essential oils into small particles and then it diffuse them into the air and the environment. It is really the best idea that you buy good quality of essential oils rather than lower grade oils, that you could be inhaling chemicals that they are mixed with into your lungs.

With the best quality you are breathing in 100% pure essential oils. When it comes to diffusers you will find that there are many styles to choose from. Using a diffuser to get your essential oils is one of the best ways to do this. Once you inhale the essential oils from the air they will go straight to your brain as well as other parts of your body which regulates and moderates the body functions.

Some Benefits of Using Essential Oils

Some of the benefits you will gain from using essential oils are the following:

- You will gain a feeling of peace and well being
- A fragrant wonderful smelling home environment
- Help with reducing stress and improving mood
- Purifying the air of germs
- A great booster to the immune system

There are four categories for diffusers: nebulizing, ultrasonic, evaporative, and heat. Often essential oils are diluted by using a carrier oil such as sweet almond oil, grape seed oil, olive oil, coconut oil etc. I hope that you and your loved ones will enjoy the recipes for essential oils to be used with your diffuser. Enjoy the smell of well-being!

Collection of Essential Oil Diffuser Recipes

This first blend of essential oils for your diffuser will have you feeling good and happy.

1. Sunshine Blend
Ingredients:

- one drop of Bergamot

- three drops of Lemon

- three drops of Grapefruit

- four drops of Orange

Directions:

Add oils and begin diffusing!

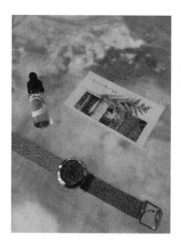

2. Forest of Citrus Blend
Ingredients:

- three drops of Lime

- three drops of Lemon

- two drops of White Fir

- one drop of Bergamot

- three drops of Orange

Directions:

Add your oils and enjoy that lively smell of citrus oils drifting through your home.

In the picture above is a diffuser bracelet!

3. Bye Bye Allergies
Ingredients:

- three drops of Lavender

- three drops of Lemon

- three drops of Peppermint

Directions:

Blend and diffuse this oil blend and enjoy no more allergy irritations.

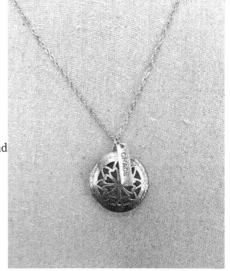

4. Calm & Relaxing Blend
Ingredients:

- 20 drops of Orange

- 20 drops of Marjoram

- 10 drops of White Chamomile (Roman)

- 8 drops of Blue Chamomile (German)

- 20 drops of Lavender

Directions:

Combine all of your oils add the drops of oil onto water usually on top of the diffuser. Now sit back and enjoy this wonderful aroma that is going to leave the atmosphere of your home feeling calm and relaxed.

In the picture is a diffuser necklace!

5. Feeling Focused Blend
Ingredients:

- three drops of Balance
- three drops of Vetiver
- four drops of Frankincense

Directions:

Blend and diffuse your oils this will help you at times when you need to stay focused such as studying for your exams!

6. Romance in the Air Blend
Ingredients:

- six drops of Orange
- six drops of Cassia

Directions:

Blend your oils and then diffuse them sending off an aroma that may get you in the mood for love!

7. *Workout Boost Blend*

Ingredients:

- three drops of Grapefruit
- three drops of Peppermint
- three drops of Slim and Sassy

Directions:

Blend your oils together and diffuse this is blend is going to give you that added boost you need to make it through your workout!

8. Stress Be Gone Blend
Ingredients:

- two drops of Marjoram
- three drops of Ylang Ylang
- three drops of Clary Sage
- six drops of Lavender

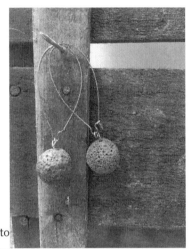

Directions:

Blend and diffuse these oils and begin to feel the stress of life be lifted from your shoulders!

Above in the picture are diffuser earrings!

9. Easy Breath Blend
Ingredients:

- two drops of Peppermint
- three drops of Eucalyptus
- three drops of Breathe

Directions:

Blend your oils and diffuse this will help you to breathe easier on those days that you are having a hard time breathing, inhale and breath easy!

10. Emotional Wellness & Healing Blend
Ingredients:

- three drops of Frankincense
- two drops of Cypress
- three drops of Bergamot
- two drops of Orange

Directions:

Blend your oils and diffuse then begin to breath in and start your emotional healing.

11. Macho Man's Blend
Ingredients:

- three drops of White Fir
- two drops of Cypress
- three drops of Wintergreen

- one drop of lime

Directions:

Blend and diffuse and look out ladies here comes the man of romance "Macho Man."

12. Breath of Happiness Blend

Ingredients:

- six drops of Citrus Bliss
- six drops of Elevation

Directions:

Blend and diffuse your oils and sit back and feel your spirits be lifted with each inhale you do!

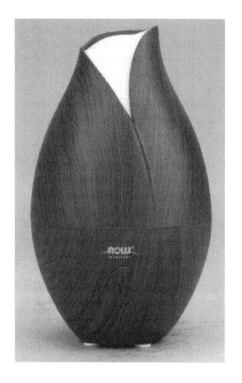

13. Finding Serenity Blend

Ingredients:

- two drops of Vanilla Bean Extract
- one drop of Sandalwood
- one drop of Ylang Ylang
- two drops of Roman Chamomile
- two drops of Sweet Marjoram
- two drops of Lavender

Directions:

Blend your essential oil and diffuse and sit back in your favorite chair and enjoy the surrounding feeling you have of peace and tranquillity with each inhale you have.

14. Invigorating Citrus Blend

Ingredients:

- one drop of Vanilla Absolute
- one drop of Clementine
- one drop of Tangerine
- one drop of Bergamot
- one drop of Mandarin
- one drop of Grapefruit
- one drop of Lemon
- one drop of Orange

Directions:

After you have blended and diffused your oils you are going to feel yourself becoming very energized and filled with the invigorating citrus blend of oils—giving you that extra boost that you needed!

15. Pleasant Dream Blend

Ingredients:

- eight drops of Vetiver

- twenty drops of Lavender

Directions:

Blend this recipe with fractionated coconut oil and put into a roller bottle and apply before you are ready to go to sleep. Before you know it you will not have insomnia but you will instead be having pleasant dreams!

16. Stamina Blend

Ingredients:

- five drops of Orange

- five drops of Peppermint

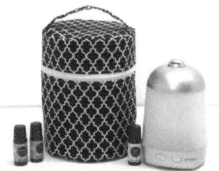

Directions:

Blend and diffuse your oils, you are soon going to feel that you have the stamina and energy you need to get what you need to get done on that day—you have been boosted!

17. Feelings of Joy & Gratitude Blend
Ingredients:

- three drops of Geranium
- three drops of White Fir
- four drops of Orange
- four drops of Bergamot

Directions:

Blend your oils and diffuse then sit back and breath in the air and allow your mood to change to one that is full of joy and gratitude for what you have in your life—enjoy this sense of calm and serenity!

18. Natural Bug Repellent
Ingredients:

- one drop of Rosemary
- two drops of Eucalyptus
- one drop of Thyme
- one drop of Melaleuca
- four drops of Lemongrass

Directions:

Blend your oils and diffuse them and watch the bugs fly in the opposite direction!

19. Big Boys Blend
Ingredients:

- two drops of Wintergreen

- two drops of Cypress EO

- four drops of White Fir

Directions:

Blend and diffuse these oils and take a walk back into the days when cavemen walked the earth! If you want that masculine kind of aroma then this blend is for you.

20. Smell the Flowers Blend
Ingredients:

- one drop of Roman Chamomile

- one drop of Lavender

- two drops of Geranium

- one drop of Clary Sage

Directions:

Just blend and diffuse these oils and breath in and feel like you are smack dab in the middle of a wonderful botanical garden totally surrounded with sweet smelling flowers!

21. Respiratory Boost Blend
Ingredients:

- one drop of Eucalyptus
- one drop of Rosemary
- two drops of Peppermint
- one drop of Lime
- two drops of Lemon

Directions:

Blend your oils and diffuse them and find that you will wake up feeling that you can breathe easy once again.

22. Feeling Sleepy Blend
Ingredients:

- one drop of Ylang Ylang
- two drops of Patchouli
- two drops of Lavender
- one drop of Bergamot

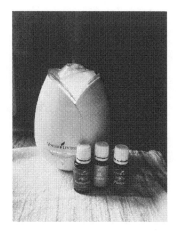

Directions:

Blend and diffuse your oils and lay back and get ready to nod off for a wonderful and peaceful night of sleep!

23. Seasonal Blend

Ingredients:

- two drops of Peppermint

- two drops of Lemongrass

- two drops of Lavender

Directions:

This blend will be perfect for the Spring and Summer seasons. It is a great blend that will help improve your immune system, inhale and heal!

24. Spray of Citrus Blend

Ingredients:

- one drop of Bergamot

- one drop of Grapefruit

- one drop of Wild Orange

- two drops of Lime

- two drops of Lemon

Directions:

Just blend and diffuse these oils and this will give your home a wonderful scent of happiness and cleanliness. This is a great blend to use when you are expecting company, this air of freshness will remain throughout your home.

25. Odor Blaster Blend
Ingredients:

- one drop of Cilantro
- one drop of White Fir
- two drops of Lime
- one drop of Melaleuca
- two drops of Lemon

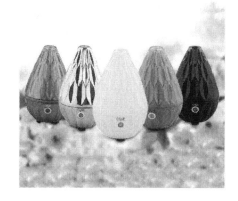

Directions:

Blend oils and diffuse, this blend will get rid of nasty odors in your home in seconds. Once you have diffused the bend no one will be able to tell that a bad odor existed just seconds before you diffused this wonderful odor blaster blend.

26. Fresh & Bright Blend
Ingredients:

- two drops of Rosemary
- two drops of Lemongrass
- two drops of Lavender

Directions:

Diffuse your oils and this wonderful blend will have your home smelling fresh and bright, it will create a welcoming atmosphere in your home.

27. Rise & Shine Blend
Ingredients:

- two drops of Wild Orange

- one drop of Lime

- two drops of Peppermint

Directions:

This blend when you diffuse it you are going to feel much more alert and on the ball. It is a great way to help get you ready to take on the day ahead! It is ideal for a cold-air diffuser you can add a small amount of water, blend and diffuse.

28. Knock Out Depression Blend
Ingredients:

- two drops of Sandalwood

- three drops of Melissa

- two drops of Geranium

- two drops of Basil

Directions:

Blend your oils and diffuse and inhale in a boost in life and exhale the depression out of your life!

29. Stress-Be-Gone Blend
Ingredients:

- five drops of Lemon
- five drops of Basil
- five drops of Rosemary
- two drops of Lime

Directions:

Blend your oils together then place the blend on a cotton ball and put into a plastic bag. Then inhale the aroma nice and deep. This will help you to open your mind and focus on whatever you are studying or working on.

30. Soothing Sore Feet Blend
Ingredients:

- two drops of Tea Tree oil
- one tablespoon of Epsom salts
- two drops of Spruce needle

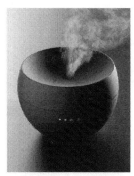

Directions:

Add the ingredients—two to three drops of oil blend. This will do you for two or three foot baths or soaks. Just add to a foot bath that is full of tepid water and blend in and soak your tender tootsies.

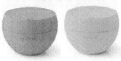

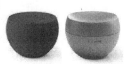

31. Remove Musty Smell Blend
Ingredients:

- two and a half teaspoons of coconut emulsifier

- 10 drops of Cedarwood

- 10 drops of Lavender

- 10 drops of Lemon

- five drops of Lime

Directions:

Add your ingredients into an amber bottle adding 50 drops with half a teaspoon of coconut emulsifier. Pour this into PET plastic spray bottle and add four ounces of water, shake well. Spray this mix onto surface in basement where you are getting unwanted odor from. Spray around your basement. You can use this in a diffuser but do not add the emulsifier and water.

32. Clothing Cedarwood Smell Blend
Ingredients:

- 15 drops of Orange

- 10 drops of Clove bud

- 40 drops of Cedarwood Atlas

Directions:

Blend these in an amber bottle. Add several drops of blend on a Terra Cotta Disc Diffuser. Allow the oil to soak in then place the disk in corner of clothing shelf. This will fill your clothing with the lovely scent of Cedarwood.

33. Refresh Carpet Blend
Ingredients:

- one quarter of a teaspoon of Litsea Cubeba
- half a teaspoon of Tangerine
- two teaspoons of Lime
- one cup of baking powder

Directions:

Mix all of the ingredients into a glass pint jar. Leave mix for 24 hours and then sprinkle over your carpet and leave on the carpet for half an hour or so then vacuum up. When you have high humidity and all the bacteria and mold could be lurking in your carpet and will make it smell badly. Add this mix to your carpet and have it smelling fresh and clean in no time! Keep any remainder of mix in a jar with tight lid in the refrigerator.

34. Body Spray Blend
Ingredients:

- 30 drops of Coconut Emulsifier
- five drops of Litsea Cubeba
- 15 drops of S'Woods
- four drops of Vanilla Absolute Pure
- two ounces of unscented base body spray

Directions:

In a two ounce PET bottle, combine your essential oils and add the emulsifier to this. Then add two ounces of unscented body spray. Shake mixture well. Spray this onto your body after you have showered, or maybe you might just want to freshen your scent up.

35. Winter Wood Blend

Ingredients:

- three drops of Wintergreen

- two drops of Cypress

- three drops of White Fir

- three drops of Cedarwood

Directions:

Blend your oils and diffuse, this smell will remind you of taking a lovely hike through a forest on a lovely winters day!

36. Holiday Mix Blend

Ingredients:

- two drops of Wild Orange

- three drops of Cassia

Directions:

Blend your oils and diffuse and inhale the spirit of the holidays!

37. Spicy Cider Blend
Ingredients:

- three drops of Ginger

- four drops of Cinnamon

- four drops of Wild Orange

Directions:

Blend and diffuse this blend will really help you to become calm and grounded!

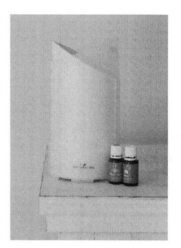

38. Under the Weather Blend
Ingredients:

- three drops of Lemon

- two drops of Frankincense

- three drops of OnGuard Blend

Directions:

This is a great blend of oils to diffuse that will help battle the germs and will boost your mood!

39. Floral Rush Blend

Ingredients:

- four drops of Idaho Balsam Fir

- five drops of Frankincense

- 15 drops of Royal Hawaiian Sandalwood

- 20 drops of Jasmine

Directions:

Blend and diffuse this wonderful blend that will give you a lovely flowery rush of smell all around you!

40. Spiritual Boost Blend

Ingredients:

- ten drops of Hinoki

- six drops of Myrrh

- one drop of Juniper

- six drops of Citrus Fresh

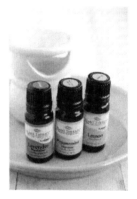

Directions:

Blend your oils and diffuse and begin to feel your spirits being lifted with each inhale of this comforting blend of essential oils!

Conclusion

I hope that you have read this book and are now ready and waiting to get busy trying out this collection of essential oil diffuser recipes. I hope that you will enjoy putting these to good use in bringing a sense of calm and comfort into your home environment through the use of essential oils via a diffuser. Of course once you become more familiar with all the different kinds of essential oils you can even begin to experiment making up your own blends using your favorite oils.

I wish you great pleasure and satisfaction in trying this collection of essential oil blends. Just think how nice it will be when you walk into your home and it smells of a wonderful blend of essential oils that make it so much more a zone of comfort in this busy world we live in! There is nothing better to going home from a busy day to be greeted at the door by a wonderful blend of essential oils aromatherapy!

FREE Bonus Reminder

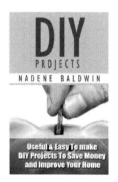

If you have not grabbed it yet, please go ahead and download your special bonus report *"DIY Projects. 13 Useful & Easy To Make DIY Projects To Save Money & Improve Your Home!"*

Simply Click the Button Below

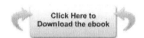

OR **Go to This Page**

http://diyhomecraft.com/free

BONUS #2: More Free & Discounted Books

Do you want to receive more Free & Discounted Books?

We have a mailing list where we send out our new Books when they go free or with a discount on Kindle. Click on the link below to sign up for Free & Discount Book Promotions.

=> Sign Up for Free & Discount Book Promotions <=

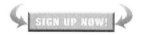

OR Go to this URL

http://zbit.ly/1WBb1Ek

Made in the USA
Las Vegas, NV
07 February 2022

43357941R00020